Table of Contents

Introduction

As we head into this shiny new millennium, we're repeatedly reminded of the coming together of East and West. That fusion no doubt has something to do with the satellite television programming that now beams in shows from diverse cultures, with the increased availability of books and music from faraway places that merely a generation or two ago were not within reach, and, of course, with the way we now connect with people across time and space through the Internet and other telecommunications improvements.

YOGA

In short, the world has become a much, much smaller place. Indeed, when Marshall McLuhan, the celebrated Canadian educator, philosopher and scholar, coined the term *Global Village*, even he probably didn't envision so much happening, so quickly, so soon.

Although the wave of information that now crisscrosses our tiny planet is something that has its roots in ancient history, it is now experiencing a burgeoning in the West that continues to gain momentum with each passing year.

And yoga has not escaped this worldwide phenomenon. Whether it's at a local YMCA or a lush spiritual retreat in the Everglades, yoga is establishing itself as a mainstay in Western culture, indeed, in global culture.

And yet, many people are reluctant to experience the physical, emotional, and psychological health benefits of yoga, and there is really only one major reason for this: misinformation.

Although many people might truly enjoy yoga and find it to be the side-effect-free answer to a lot of their emotional and physical ailments, they just don't know enough about the subject to take that first step.

Moreover, despite considerable evidence to the contrary, the notion seems to persist that yoga is a religious following, and that to experience its many health benefits somehow obliges one to renounce their faith or, worse, run away to some commune and eat tofu in between chanting sessions.

Although, yes, if you'd like to go to a retreat and enjoy tofu and chanting, that's probably possible. (Almost anything is possible, as long as it's legal and people want to do it, right?)

Yet that vision of yoga – people with shaved heads handing out flowers to strangers at the airport – is by no means the overall picture. Yoga is really a very simple, accessible, and, in many countries around the world, ordinary thing to do.

In that light, this book was created with one goal in mind: to demystify yoga for you, and provide you with a clear, simple, and enjoyable introduction to this form of exercise.

If you've never been exposed to any kind of yoga (except for what you might have seen on television), this book will be especially beneficial for you.

But even if you have tried some kinds of yoga (maybe a friend dragged you to a class at the local recreation center all those years ago), this book might reawaken your interest in the subject and reattach you back to a system of body movement and mind focus that has been used in ancient lands for a millennium.

This book is divided into four sections:

☑ **What is Yoga?**

☑ **Why is Yoga Beneficial?**

☑ **Different Kinds of Yoga**

☑ **Yoga Equipment & Accessories**

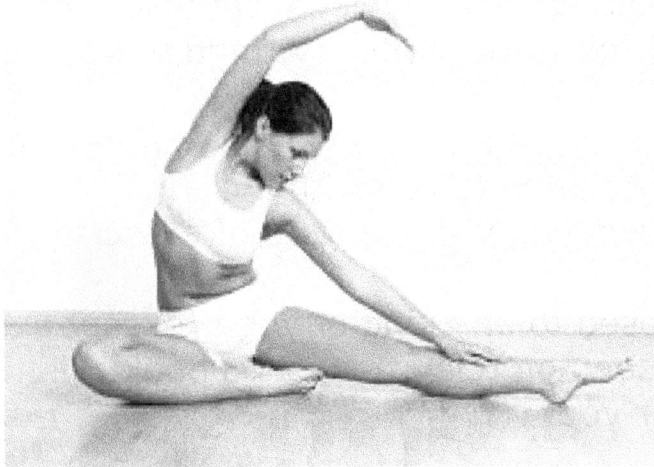

As you read through these sections, please bear in mind that there is absolutely *no* attempt here, directly or indirectly (or in any other way possible) to endorse or promote any religious view. This is because the view of this book is same view that is held by the world's foremost authorities on yoga: that it is *not* a religion. It does not have a dogma.

Although there many different schools and streams of yoga, they have all managed to coexist peacefully because, for the most part, yoga is not evangelical, which means it does not seek to spread itself as part of its mission.

Please note that the statement above in no way criticizes or comments on evangelical orders, such as Evangelical Christianity. The point here is simply that the overwhelming majority of yoga movements do not consider *spreading* yoga to be a tenet of its identity.

Yet, while the yoga that is described in this book (and experienced in most of the world) is *not* a religion, it *does* fir seamlessly into many people's existing religious framework.

In other words, if you are a Catholic, a Protestant, a Muslim, a Jew, a Sikh, or anything else and identify yourself as being a part of *any* faith at all, yoga doesn't ask you to replace that faith with someone else, or offer you a competing or contradictory view of what you already believe.

So please remember: yoga, as it is discussed and promoted in this book (and in virtually every yoga book worth reading) is *not* a religion.

As we'll begin to understand in the next section of this book, yoga is really nothing more, and nothing less, than harassing the power of human attention and using it to benefit the body and mind. It is an approach to life, here and now.

What is Yoga?

What was I looking for that night in Bombay? The same thing I had been looking for as long as I can remember. The same thing all of us seek in one way or another. The "answer" to life, whatever that might mean. The "truth." The reason for living, dying, or being "here" at all.

- Beryl Bender Birch

Yoga can seem like a complicated concept, or, at the very least, a dizzying array of physical manipulations that turn seemingly happy-looking human beings into happy-looking human *pretzels*.

Or even more disconcerting, as we have alluded to in the Introduction, a stereotype does exist in places where the term yoga is synonymous with *cult*, or some kind of archaic spiritual belief that compels one to quit their job, sell their house, and go live in the middle of nowhere.

In actual fact, Yoga is a very basic thing, and if you've had the opportunity to visit a country where it has been established for generations – India, Japan, China, and others – it's really rather, well, *ordinary*.

The practice of yoga came to the West back in 1893 when one of India's celebrated gurus, Swami Vivekananda, was welcomed at the World Fair in Chicago. He is now known for having *sparked* the West's interest in yoga.

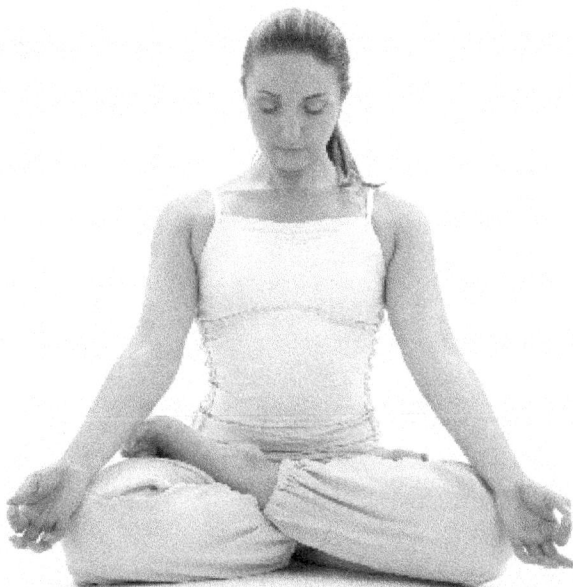

Literally, the word yoga comes from the Sanskrit term *Yug*, which means: "to yoke, bind, join, or direct one's attention." At the same time, yoga can also imply concepts such as *fusion, union*, and *discipline.*

The sacred scriptures of Hinduism (an ancient belief system from India that has a global presence) also defines yoga as "unitive discipline," the kind of discipline that, according to experts Georg Feuerstein and Stephan Bodian in their book *Living Yoga*, leads to inner and outer union, harmony and joy.

In essence, yoga is most commonly understood as *conscious living*, of tapping into one's inner potential for happiness (what Sankrit refers to as *ananda*).

What Yoga Isn't

Sometimes it's helpful to understand things by what they *aren't*, especially when dealing with a topic, like yoga, that is quite easily misunderstood.

Authors and yoga scholars Feuerstein and Bodian help us understand yoga by telling us what it is NOT:

- × **Yoga is NOT calisthenics (marked by the headstand, the lotus posture or some pretzel-like pose). Although it is true that yoga involves many**

postures – especially in hatha yoga – these are
only intended to make people get in touch with
their inner feelings.

× Yoga is NOT a system of meditation – or a religion
– the way many people are misled to believe.
Meditation is only part of the whole process of
bringing ourselves into the realm of the spiritual.

The Essence of Yoga

Virtually all yogic science and philosophy contends that a
human being is but a fragment of an enormous universe,
and when this human being learns to "communion" with this
vastness, then he/she attains union with something that is
bigger than him/her. This attachment, or *tapping into
something bigger,* thus enables one to walk the true path of
happiness. By flowing along with the force, the individual is
able to discover truth.

And with truth comes *realization*, but to attain realization,
our words, thoughts and deeds must be based on truth.
People attend courses on yoga and go to studios to learn
new techniques in yoga, but yoga teacher Tim Miller said

that "true yoga begins when [you] leave the studio, it's all about being awake and being mindful of your actions."

Yoga and Physical Health

Yoga does not see a distinction between the body and the mind, and this is an understanding that Western psychology

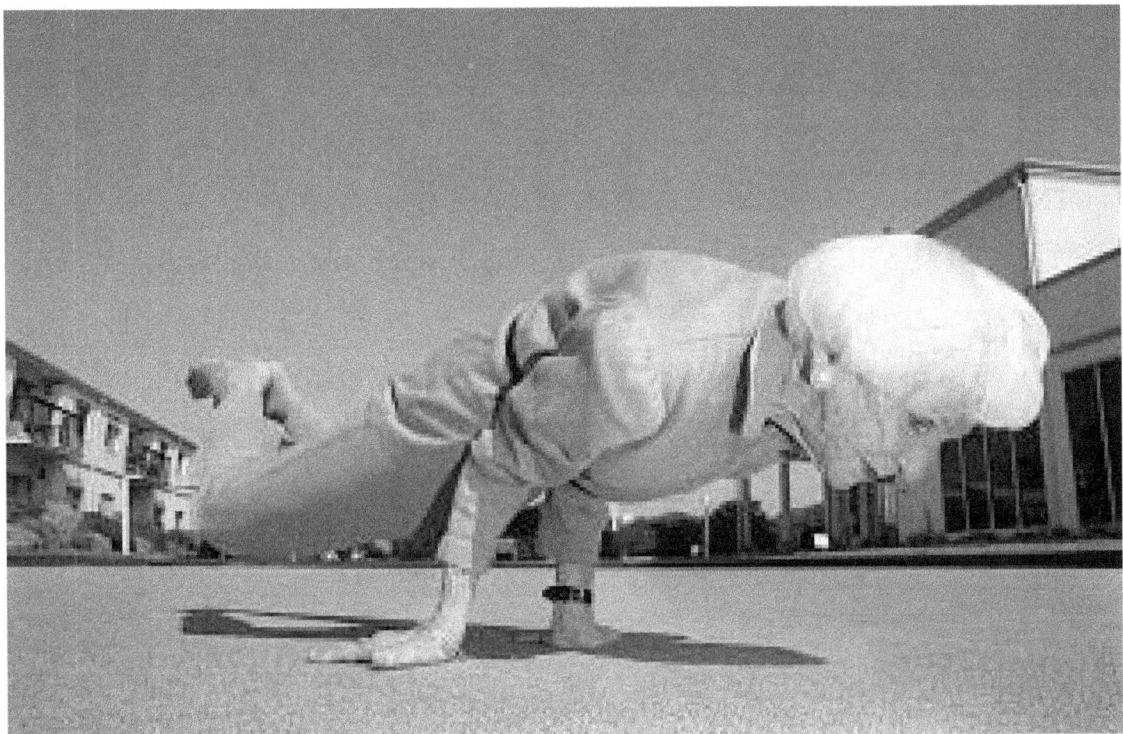

has also concluded for many years now (the link between mental health and physical health, and vice versa).

If you've come to this book looking to understand yoga as a means to help your body heal or improve, then please don't worry, **you've come to the right place.**

Yoga is indeed a process that involves releasing blocked tension and energy in the body, and helping make the muscles, tendons, joints, ligaments, and all other components work to their utmost potential.

Yoga believes that human beings are optimally designed, by nature to be flexible and agile, and stiffness and lack of mobility arrive only when the body is unhealthy or out of alignment.

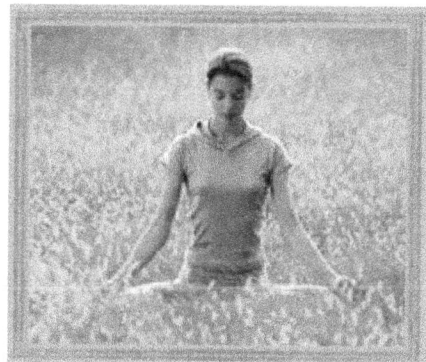

Therefore, countless people have found themselves in a yoga class, or on a yoga mat at home in front of a yoga video or DVD, in the hopes of improving their physical health, and maybe you are one of them. If that's the case, *keep reading!*

There are proven physical benefits of yoga, which include:

- ✓ **increased flexibility and range of motion**

- ✓ **reduced pain in joints and muscles**

- ✓ **stronger immune system**

- ✓ **stronger lung capacity and therefore higher quality respiration**

- ✓ **increased metabolism (which can lead to weight loss)**

- ✓ **higher quality of sleep (especially due to improved breathing and a more oxygenated body)**

Given that certain yoga practices require postures to be mastered, yoga has always helped promote the body's flexibility; it also helps in lubricating the joints, ligaments and tendons. Yoga detoxifies by increasing the flow of blood to various parts of the body. It helps tone and invigorates muscles that have grown flaccid and weak.

So please do keep in mind that although yoga is often discussed in terms of its *mental* approach, there are clear and <u>proven physical benefits</u> that are a part of this approach.

Therefore, if weight loss is your goal, or the ability to shovel the snow in winter without having your back ache for days, then yoga is as viable an option to you as it is for the stressed-out corporate executive who needs to find a strategy for coping with the craziness if her busy life.

> *Yoga is thus just not twisting the body to perform certain asanas or postures but balancing the mind and body, making it more receptive to the universal life force pouring from the Supreme Self. Hence, be truthful, do your duty and love all, along with a few asanas daily to keep yourself on the path of evolution.*
>
> *Meena Om, in Yoga – Beyond the Body and Mind.*

Why is Yoga Beneficial?

As we've repeatedly pointed out in this book (and probably started to bore you with, sorry), yoga is *not* a religion. It *can* be religious if one wants it to be, and it can co-exist with an existing religious belief. But yoga itself is not religious in the sense that it focuses on belief or faith.

Yoga is a science, and indeed, in many places in the world (such as India) it is referred to as a science. This is not mere playing with words, it truly is approached as a science, which means that it is understood in terms of the scientific method.

Yogic science seeks to verify cause and effect and build principles based upon objective observations. Indeed, in many places in the world, to be a yogic master of any credibility, one must be highly educated in the sciences, including physics and the biological sciences.

This discussion on yoga as *science* is important for us to have here, because it allows us to sensibly ask the question: What are the benefits of yoga? After all, if yoga is a faith or a belief, then asking this question isn't fair, because it's one that yoga cannot answer in terms that we can objectively understand.

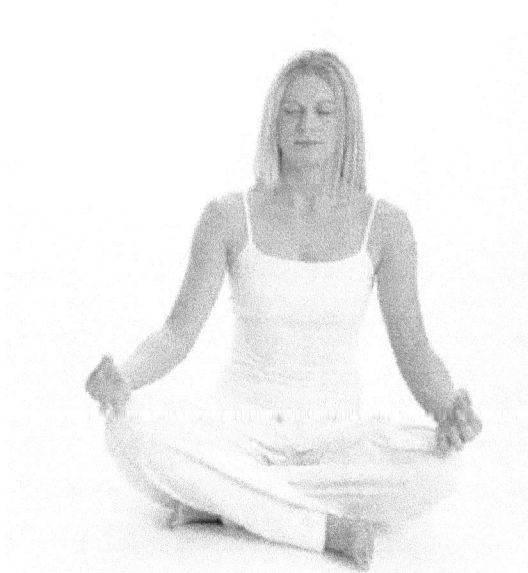

Yet yoga is a science, as empirical and pragmatic as kinesiology or exercise science, which seeks to understand how the body acts and *reacts* to changes in the internal physical environment. And before we are asked to consider experiencing yoga for ourselves, each of us has a right to ask the basic question, "*Why should I bother doing this yoga thing?*"

Indeed, while the experience of yoga cannot be reduced to words – just as reading a book on preparing for a marathon isn't going to actually physically prepare you to run a marathon – the goals and principles of yoga can easily be discussed.

Here's the Mayo Clinic's take on the benefits of meditation:

> Meditation is used by people who are perfectly healthy as a means of stress reduction. But if you have a medical condition that's worsened by stress, you might find the practice valuable in reducing the stress-related effects of allergies, asthma, chronic pain and arthritis, among others.
>
> Yoga involves a series of postures, during which you pay special attention to your breathing — exhaling during certain movements and inhaling with others. You can approach yoga as a way to promote physical flexibility, strength and endurance or as a way to enhance your spirituality.

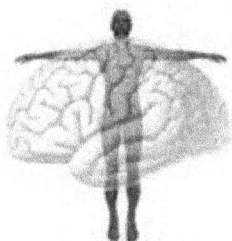

The Mind-Body Connection

helps us understand, yoga is centered on the mind-body connection. This mind-body harmony is achieved through three things:

> postures (*asanas*)

> proper breathing (*pranayama*)

> meditation

Mind and body draw inspiration and guidance from the combined practices of *asanas*, breathing, and meditation. As people age (to yogis, aging is an artificial condition), our bodies become susceptible to toxins and poisons (caused by environmental and poor dietary factors).

Yoga helps us through a cleaning process, turning our bodies into a well-synchronized and well-oiled piece of machinery.

Physical Benefits

By harmonizing these three principles, the benefits of yoga are attained. And just what are these benefits?

⇨ **equilibrium in the body's central nervous system**

⇨ **decrease in pulse**

⇨ **respiratory and blood pressure rates**

⇨ **cardiovascular efficiency**

⇨ **gastrointestinal system stabilization**

⇨ **increased breath-holding time**

⇨ **improved dexterity skills.**

⇨ **Improved balance**

⇨ **Improved depth perception**

Psychological Benefits

As noted above, yoga also delivers an array of psychological benefits, and in fact, this is a very common reason people begin practicing it in the first place. Perhaps the most frequently mentioned psychological benefit of yoga is an improved ability to manage *stress*. Yoga diminishes an individual's levels of anxiety, depression, and lethargy, thus enabling him/her to focus on what's spiritual and important: achieving balance and happiness.

Supporting a Healthy Lifestyle

There is some very interesting psychology behind this that students of Western thinkers (e.g., Freud, Jung, Fromm, etc.) will find familiar and, indeed, quite rational. When an individual *decides* to be happy, something within that person activates a kind of *will* or *awareness*. This

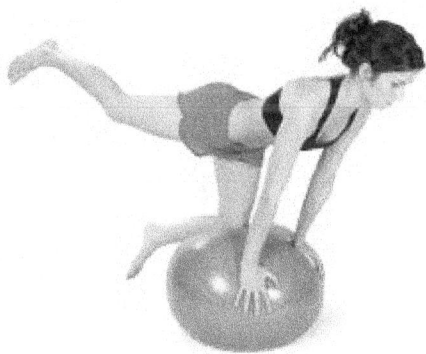

awareness begins to observe the jungle of negative thoughts that are swimming constantly through the mind.

Rather than attacking each of these thoughts – because that would be an *unending* struggle – yoga simply advises the individual to watch that struggle, and through that watching, the stress will diminish (because it becomes exposed and thus unfed by the unconscious, unobserving mind).

At the same time, as an individual begins to reduce his or her level of internal negativity, subsequent *external negative behaviors* begin to fall of their own accord, habits such as excessive drinking, emotional overeating, and engaging in behaviors that, ultimately, lead to unhappiness and suffering.

With this being said, it would be an overstatement to imply that practicing yoga is the *easy way* to, say, quit smoking, or to start exercising regularly. If that were the case, yoga would be ideal. Yoga simply says that, based on rational and scientific cause and effect relationships that have been observed for *centuries*, when a person begins to feel good inside, they naturally tend to behave in ways that enhance and promote this feeling of inner wellness.

As such, although smoking (for example) is an addiction and the body will react to the lessening of addictive ingredients such as tar and tobacco (just to name two of many), yoga will *help* the process. It will help provide the individual with the strength and *logic* that they need in order to discover that smoking actually doesn't make them feel good.

In fact, once they start observing how they feel, they'll notice without doubt that instead of feeling good, smoking actually makes one feel quite bad inside. It's harder to breathe, for one thing.

Now, this book isn't an anti-smoking book, and if you've struggled with quitting smoking, please don't be offended by any of this; there is **no attempt here at all** to imply that quitting smoking is *easy*, or just a matter of *willpower*.

Scientists have proven that there is a true physical addiction that is in place, alongside an emotional addiction that can be just as strong, perhaps even stronger.

The point here is simply to help you understand that yoga can help a person make conscious living choices that promote healthy and *happy* living. This can include:

- ✓ **quitting smoking**

- ✓ **reducing excess drinking**

- ✓ **eating healthier**

- ✓ **getting more sleep**

- ✓ **reducing stress at work (and everywhere else for that matter)**

- ✓ **promoting more harmonious relationships all around**

Please remember: Yoga *doesn't* promise anyone that these things will simply *happen* overnight. At most, yoga is the light that shows you how messy things in the basement really are, and once that light is on, it becomes much more straightforward – not to mention efficient and time effective – to clean things up.

Emotional Benefits

Yoga has also been hailed for its special ability to help people eliminate feelings of hostility and inner resentment. As a result of eliminating these toxic emotions, the doorway to self-acceptance and self-actualization opens.

Pain Management Benefits

Pain management is another benefit of yoga. Since pain and chronic pain are conditions that affect all of us at some point, understanding the positive link between yoga and pain management could be invaluable.

It can also be *financially* valuable, since the pain medication industry is a multi-billion dollar marketplace and many people, especially as they age, find that their insurance or government coverage won't cover some pharmaceutical and over-the-counter pain relief medications.

Yoga is believed to reduce pain by helping the brain's pain center regulate the gate-controlling mechanism located in the spinal cord and the secretion of natural painkillers in the body.

Breathing exercises used in yoga can also reduce pain. Because muscles tend to relax when you exhale, lengthening the time of exhalation can help produce relaxation and reduce tension.

Awareness of breathing helps to achieve calmer, slower respiration and aid in relaxation and pain management. Yoga's inclusion of relaxation techniques and meditation can also help reduce pain. Part of the effectiveness of yoga in reducing pain is due to its focus on self-awareness.

This self-awareness can have a protective effect and allow for early preventive action.

Real People, Real Benefits

> Bikram Yoga has helped manage my diabetes unbelievably. I have curtailed my insulin injections by 50%. I have lost 30 pounds, completely lost the desires to smoke, drink alcohol and eat junk food. I even wrote a book on how it saved my life called, No More Diabetes, How Yoga Saved my Life.
>
> - John Spanek

Different Kinds of Yoga

It's funny to look at it this way, but one of the things that has promoted the spread of yoga in the West is the same thing that can sometimes prevent someone from truly exploring it and therefore experiencing its health benefits. This thing is *variety*.

Sometimes when there is only one of something – such as one idea, or one language, or one *anything* – it's hard for that thing to spread outside of those who abide by it, agree with it, or simply want it to continue existing.

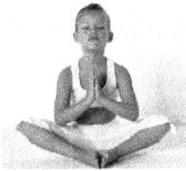

Yet when there are *multiple* ideas and concepts, the chances of it spreading increase; there are just more people out there who will be able to access it, talk about it, and indeed, make it a part of their lives.

What does this have to do with yoga? Well, there are many different *types* of yoga, and the reason for this, as we initially discussed, is that yoga isn't a religion, it's an approach to being alive. As such, it's very agile and flexible (no pun intended) and carries well across cultural, country, and religious boundaries.

Thanks to its diversity and different facets and types, yoga has spread very swiftly through the Western world over the past 110 years or so, and is spreading faster now than ever before (many western companies will now pay for yoga classes as part of an enhanced health benefits program).

Yet this very diversity has led to some confusion, and people who have been exposed to one kind of yoga might accidentally think that they've *seen it all*. This is more worrisome, of course, when one has been exposed to a kind of yoga that – for whatever reason – they did not like, or perhaps, weren't quite ready for (just as how some people might turn away from a fitness program if they aren't in the right frame of mind to see it through).

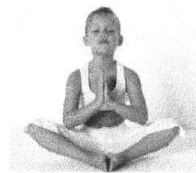

So if you've experienced yoga, or seen it on television, read about it in a newspaper, or overheard a friend or colleague talk about it, then please be aware that there's a *very good*

chance that you haven't been exposed to all that there is (which is wonderful, because it means that this next section will be very interesting and informative for you!).

Six Major Types

Yogic scholars Feuerstein and Bodian note six major types of yoga. In no particular order, they are:

> hatha yoga

> raja yoga

> karma yoga

> bhakti yoga

> jnana yoga

> tantra yoga

Let's look at each one of these in turn.

Hatha Yoga

Graham Ledgerwood, who has been teaching yoga and mysticism for over 30 years, says that hatha yoga is practiced in the West mostly for health and vitality, and is the most popular in Western society.

Ha is a Sanskrit term meaning sun, so *hatha yoga* according to Ledgerwood is a "*marvelous means of exercising, stretching, and freeing the body so it can be a healthy, long-lived, and vital instrument of the mind and soul.*"

Perfecting the postures in hatha yoga has two objectives:

1. Meditating.

People need at least one posture that they can be totally comfortable with for a long period of time. The more postures you can master, the better you are able to cultivate deeper meditation techniques.

2. Renewing body's energies for optimum health.

Raja Yoga

Similar to classical yoga, raja yoga is considered the "royal path" to unifying the mind and body. Raja yoga is considered by some to be a rather difficult form of yoga, because it seeks enlightenment through direct control and mastery of the mind.

People who can concentrate well and enjoy meditation are best suited for raja yoga. This type – or branch – of yoga has 8 limbs:

⇨ **moral discipline**   ⇨ **sensory inhibition**

⇨ **self-restraint**   ⇨ **concentration**

⇨ **posture**   ⇨ **meditation**

⇨ **breath control**   ⇨ **ecstasy**

Karma Yoga

Karma yoga involves selfless action. The word karma itself means action – all actions that come from the individual beginning from his birth until his death. Most important, karma is the path to *doing the right thing*. Hence the practice of karma yoga means giving up the ego to serve God and humanity.

Karma yoga comes from the teachings of the *Bhagavad Vita*, which is sometimes respectfully referred to as "the New Testament of Hinduism." Service to God through serving others is the foundation of Karma Yoga.

Bhakti Yoga

Sri Swami Sivananda says:

> *Mark how love develops. First arises faith. Then follows attraction and after that adoration. Adoration leads to suppression of mundane desires. The result is single-mindedness and satisfaction. Then grow attachment and supreme love towards God.*
>
> *In this type of highest Bhakti all attraction and attachment which one has for objects of enjoyment are transferred to the only dearest object, God. This leads the devotee to an eternal union with his Beloved and culminates in oneness.*

Bhakti yoga is thus seen as *divine love*. As a force of attraction, Swami Nikhilananda and Sri Ramakrishna Math say that love operates on three levels:

1. material   **2. human**   **3. spiritual**

These two yogis further explain that love is a creative power, and this creative power pushes us to seek joy and immortality.

In their own elegant and precise words:

> Love based upon intellectual attraction is more impersonal
> and enduring... It is a matter of common observation that
> the more intellectually developed the life of a person is, the
> less he takes pleasure in the objects of the senses.

Jnana Yoga

Jnana yoga is the path to wisdom. Graham Ledgerwood defines jnana as "emptying out" the mind and soul of delusions so that individuals can be attuned to reality, releasing all thoughts and emotions until the individual is transformed and enlightened.

Jnana yoga is one of the four main paths that lead directly to self-realization (philosophy of *advaita vedanda*). By crushing the obstacles of ignorance, the student of jnana yoga experiences God.

Concepts such as discernment and discrimination are highly regarded in jnana yoga, where the student or devotee identifies himself as separate from the components of his environment. "Neti-neti" is also a principle inherent in jnana yoga. Literally, it means "not this, not this" and by removing objects around, what's left is just YOU and only you.

Tantra Yoga

A seventh type of yoga that many people have heard about, and indeed, are quite curious about, is *tantra yoga*.

Tantra yoga is considered by some to be most Oriental of all yoga branches. It is often misunderstood as consisting exclusively of sexual rituals. It involves *more* than sex; it is the path of self-transcendence through ritual means, one of which is just consecrated sexuality. Some tantric schools actually recommend a celibate lifestyle after a certain point.

Tantra literally means "expansion." A tantra devotee expands all his levels of consciousness so he/she can reach out to the Supreme Reality. Tantra yoga aims to awaken the male and female aspects within a person to trigger a spiritual awakening.

Advice for Beginners

As you now know (if you didn't know it when you started reading, that is), yoga is an interesting and ancient method of uniting the body and the mind. It has *proven* health benefits, including emotional and physical improvements.

The chances therefore are, if you're on the verge of starting a yoga program (perhaps at a local center or you've purchased a video or DVD and want to try it at home), you're excited, optimistic, and anxious to get going.

Yet it's wise to note that, before going into yoga practice, you should ask yourself some important questions. These questions don't have a *right or wrong* answer.

They are merely meant to stimulate your own thoughts and give you the mindset that you need in order to succeed as a student of yoga for the long term.

Here are the basic questions that you should ask before starting any yoga program:

⇨ **What are my reasons for starting a yoga program? Are they realistic?**

⇨ **If my yoga program involves some degree of physical strain, such as certain postures in hatha yoga, have I received medical clearance from a qualified and certified health professional to ensure that I don't injure myself?**

⇨ **Are my goals for pursuing a yoga program (or *programs*) clear and positive? Do I know what I want to achieve?**

⇨ **Am I prepared to commit the time necessary to really get the most of out of my yoga experience?**

⇨ **Are there people around me who might negatively try and talk me out (or *mock* me out) of pursuing this path of personal development? Should I either avoid such people, or ask them to respect what I'm choosing to do?**

Please note that these are just basic questions, and this isn't an exhaustive list. The point here is really that you should be clear and confident about your choice of experiencing yoga.

And remember, please: there are many different kinds of yoga, and many different kinds of *yoga instructors*. Most of them are great, a handful of them may be well-intentioned, but may lack some of the foundation that they need in order to teach.

> **Remember always: No yoga instructor that you work with should *ever* humiliate you, degrade you, insult you, or make you feel inferior.**

If you encounter the 1 in 1,000 who has not yet achieved the personal development that he/she needs in order to effectively teach, then remember: There are always other teachers.

The goal here is to make you happy, healthy, and confident. These criteria should be a part of all of your yoga experiences from day one.

Final Note on Consistency

For you to enjoy every benefit of your commitment to practicing yoga, please note that consistency and regularity are keys. You can't go into one session and skip three or four just because you're sore, had an unexpected engagement, or were too stressed out.

For the body *and mind* to change, you need to practice yoga consistently. Remove all obstacles, real or imagined and stay committed. Your rewards will be better health, better emotional balance, and a happier, more fulfilled life!

Yoga Equipment & Accessories

The popularity of yoga has given rise to an industry that specializes in yoga equipment, accessories and clothes. The internet is a true market place of things yoga and product lines are as varied and diverse as the many teachings and postures of yoga.

If you've ventured into your neighborhood sporting goods store, or even a department store, you've likely seen an

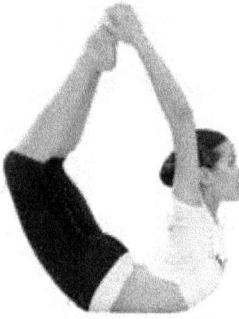

array of *yoga equipment* that features very happy and peaceful looking people sitting on a yoga mat, or using a yoga towel. Indeed, for someone interested in yoga, this is like a *kid in a candy store*. There has never been a time in the marketplace where yoga equipment was so easy to find, and indeed, so affordable.

With that being said, it can be rather confusing as to which equipment does *what*. They all seem to have such happy looking people on the packaging, how do you know what's worth investing your money in?

Well, ultimately, the answer to that important question will be determined by the kind of yoga that you want to experience, and also your own preferences.

Some people, for example, don't want to sit on a mat, they prefer the firmness of the floor. Other people find that sitting on the floor is painful and can lead to back and tailbone ache, and as such, a yoga mat is *essential*.

So, rather than prescribing here what you should buy and what you shouldn't, let's instead focus on the various neat things that you *can* easily buy, and you can use this information to help you make a wise decision.

Yoga Mats

Let's start with the famous yoga mat. Now, as a general rule (to which there will always, of course, be exceptions), be careful with the supermarket version.

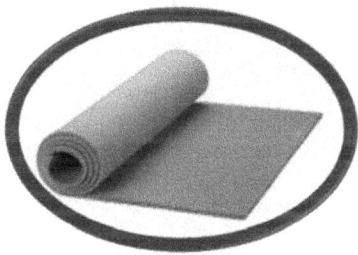

A good yoga mat has a good grip on the floor, which is important if you have to perform complicated maneuvers and postures. They typically measure about 2 feet in width, and are available in a slew of rainbow colors.

There are yoga mats to fit all levels from beginner to advanced, and you have a choice of thickness. Many yoga stores will provide mats with efficient cushioning. Yoga mats are also available for children.

Yoga Towel

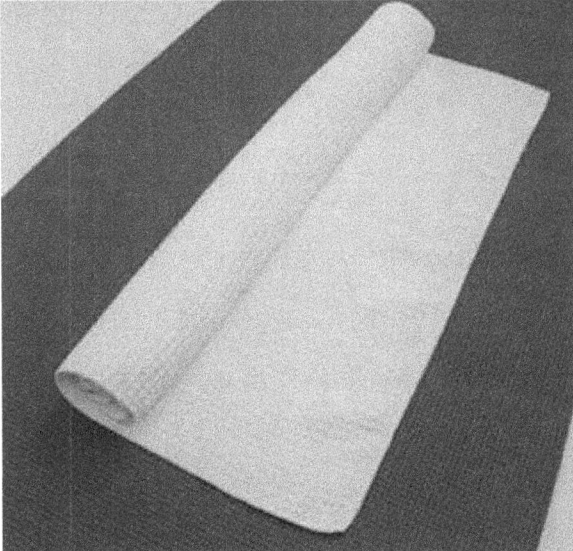

Don't forget your yoga towel. There are also skidless towels and some manufacturers make super absorbent ones – also, in what some retailers call, "chakra colors."

Yoga Bags

Yoga bags look rectangular – almost tubular – they are designed to hold your yoga mat and towel and other accessories.

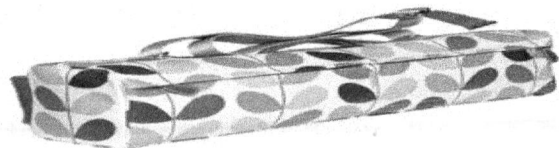

Most products have a shoulder strap and are made of different materials, nylon being a common one. There are low end yoga bags for $12, and they go up to $50, depending on make and size.

Yoga Straps

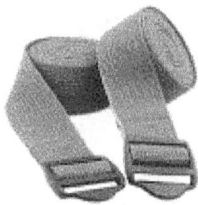

Those who do a lot of yoga flexibility routines often opt for yoga straps. These straps help them stretch their limbs, and to hold poses longer.

Yoga Sandbags and Bolsters

There are also yoga sandbags and bolsters that help your body balance and provide support as you perform your poses, stretches and positions. They are also available in many colors.

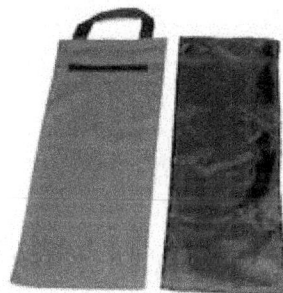

Yoga Meditation Cushions, Chairs, Benches, and Pillows

The website www.yoga.com sells kits that include what they call "cosmic meditation cushions," which are advertised as ideal for peaceful meditation. There's the backjack meditation chair (no legs) with firm upright back for support. There are also meditation benches (in different shapes) and the breathing (prayanama) pillow.

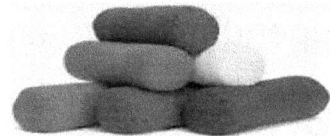

Yoga Balls

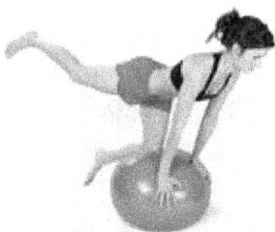

Balls are good for building strength, achieve balance and tone muscles. These fun yoga balls sell for about $25, and many dancers and physical therapists use yoga balls for a variety of movements, including backbends, restorative poses and hip openers. Many balls can hold up to 600 pounds of weight. And remember, don't forget your air pump.

Yoga Blocks

These devices look like blocks, and have a
mattress-feel to them. They're *great* for
body movement extensions.

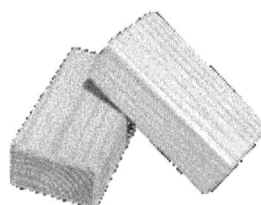

Yoga Videos/DVDs

If you're pressed for time, feel a bit shy about attending a
public yoga class, or just want to have an idea of how yoga
is practiced, yoga videos/DVDs are a great way to get
initiated into yoga.

A great advantage of yoga videos is you can watch the clips
over and over again until you've mastered the techniques
correctly.

Yoga Music

To name a few titles: Slow Music for Yoga, Tibetan Sacred Temple Music, Shiva Station, Nectar, Fragrance of the East.

There is also yoga music for trance dance and yoga flow, chants and mantras and audio books.

Yoga Clothing

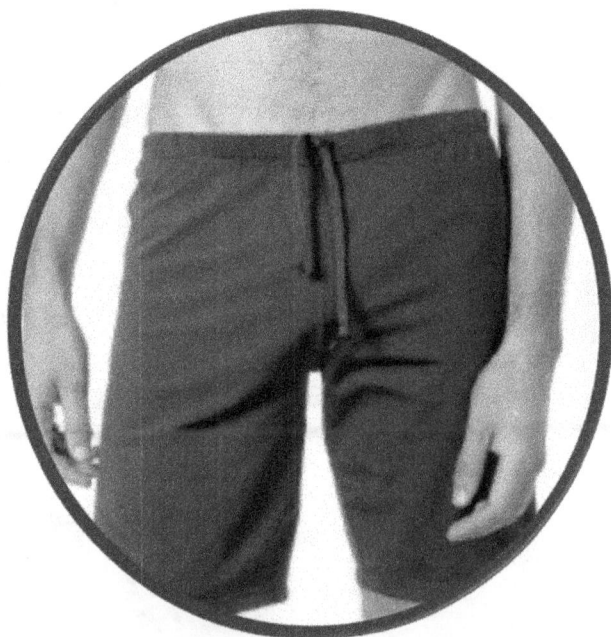

Though not mandatory for class, many yoga participants want an all-yoga attire to complement their yoga practice. Most beginners however come in a loose-fitting cotton t-shirt and comfortable leggings.

Conclusion

The journey of yoga is one that is *always* an introduction, and hence, the title of this book is a bit of a pleasant, zen-like joke. There is no *end* to yoga, it is a constant process of discovering yourself, and energizing your body to give it optimal health.

With that being said, for purely practical purposes, it's just fine to refer to something as an *introduction to yoga*, and hopefully this book has been a pleasant eye-opener for you.

Among other things, this book has ideally:

☑ **Clarified for you that yoga is *not* a religion and therefore does not request or require you to change your faith.**

☑ Helped you understand the benefits of yoga, benefits that range from physical, to emotional, to psychological improvements.

☑ Helped you understand that yoga is not an "overnight thing", but takes consistency, commitment, and routine in order to deliver all of the benefits you deserve.

☑ Helped you understand the various different kinds of yoga available to you (and *all* of these forms are available in the West, though some of the less popular one might only be centered in large urban areas).

☑ Provided you with an overview of the various equipment that you can buy (if you wish) to enhance and improve your yoga journey.

In closing – we won't say *concluding*, as there's no end to this journey – let's consider the words of Swami Akhilananda, who describes the power and joy that people who attentively follow a yogic path experience. (Please note, too, that if you don't like the usage of the word *God* in the quote below, simply replace it with something that fits your preference, the meaning and intent will remain the same.)

www.ingramcontent.com/pod-product-compliance
Lightning Source LLC
Chambersburg PA
CBHW080630030426
42336CB00018B/3146